# HOW TO MAKE TINCTURES OUT OF HERBS

By Smith J. Offor

# Table of Contents

# Introduction

**Herbal tinctures and treatments made at home.**

Herbal tinctures, also known as hydroethanolic extractions, are made from the alcoholic extract of a plant.

We can extract from plants both the water-soluble and alcohol-soluble components for a potent, well-rounded medicine using tinctures, which provide a user-friendly and fast-acting herbal medicine form. Furthermore, tinctures are extremely stable and have a very long shelf life.

Instead of having to prepare leaves, flowers, and other plant parts separately from roots, barks, and berries for teas due to their structure, tinctures let us combine and tincture every part of the plant at once. The same mixture can also be used to tincture powdered herbs in addition to cut and sifted herbs.

**Water-soluble ingredients include the following.**

Carbohydrates, Phenolics, Proteins/Amino Acids, Gum, Mucilage, Tannins, Salts, Saponins, Anthraquinones, Tannins, Saponins, and Salts are examples of chemical compounds.

The composites of alcohols:

Alkaloids, resins, glycosides, volatile oils, and tanning agents.

# A Manual for Making Tincture at Home

Both the calculation method and the traditional method can be easily used to create tinctures at home. The traditional technique is easy to follow and requires only a few basic ingredients: your herbs, alcohol, cheesecloth, and amber dropper bottles with a tight-fitting lid from a wide-mouth canning jar. If you intend to weigh your herbs using the calculation method in order to achieve a specific herb to alcohol ratio, you will also need a scale.

## How to Choose Your Liquor

To be shelf-stable, tinctures must be at least 20% alcohol by volume (ABV), or 40 proof. To capture the widest variety of both water soluble and alcohol soluble constituents, we recommend using an alcohol with an ABV of between 40 and 60 percent (80 to 120 proof). Most gin, vodka, rum, and brandies fall exactly within that range. It's a good idea to start with vodka or brandy because their flavors are still mild enough for you to taste the flavor of the herb or herbs you're using.

## The Traditional Method of Making Tinctures

A woman is adding alcohol to a container of herbs to make a tincture.

Your glass jar should be halfway full of the herb(s) of your choice.

• The jar should be fully filled with your alcohol.

• After covering the jar's mouth with a piece of parchment paper, add a metal lid.

• Shake it daily for the first week or more, as the tincture needs 4-6 weeks to macerate (infuse).

When it's time to strain, cover the jar's mouth with a layer of cheesecloth and then pour the tincture into a sizable bowl or another clean jar. You can get as much alcohol from the herbs as you can by gathering the cheesecloth and squeezing hard until the majority of the liquid is extracted from the herbs.

Either transfer your tincture to amber dropper bottles or keep it in the squeaky-clean glass jar with the tight-fitting lid (for extended storage, I advise sandwiching some brand-new parchment paper between the jar and lid).

On the label of your tincture, mention the name of the herb, how long you strained it, and how much alcohol you used.

As an example, take the arctiumlappa root tincture, January 11, 2021, 40% ABV.

The tincture should be stored in a cool, dark place.

**Calculation Process for Your Tincture.**
• To begin, weigh your herbs in grams (g) on a kitchen scale.

• A coarse coffee grinder will help you get your herbs closer to the 1:5 ratio when using "fluffy" herbs like calendula or raspberry leaf, which can be challenging to cover with the 5 parts alcohol.

• By recording the volume of alcohol you add in milliliters (mL), you can find out your final ratio.

• Once your herbs have been weighed, measure out 5 times the amount of alcohol in milliliters (mL).

For instance, 100 g of herbs will need 500 mL of alcohol.

• Add your herbs to the clean class jar, cover them with the recommended amount of alcohol, and stir to ensure that they are completely submerged.

• It's crucial to remember that all of the plant material must be submerged in alcohol, so occasionally you might need to add a little bit more.

Place the dried roots in a jar and add a clear alcohol to create a tincture.

7

The inspiration for a lifetime's interest in herbalism could come from a sip of herbal tea or a dropperful of tincture. These simple steps are frequently followed when we begin our studies, but they can occasionally be challenging when attempting to comprehend Latin binomial nomenclature, formulations, physiological actions, and historical research. The terminology used to describe different preparations is often incorrect, and tincture is one such word that is frequently used to do so.

**Herbal tinctures' intended use.**

Tinctures are concentrated herbal extracts that are made with alcohol. Although it is a rare exception, the tomes occasionally define an acetum as "a vinegar tincture. ".

## What Qualifies as a Tincture?

Concentrated herbal extracts are used in tinctures.

All extracts are not tinctures; alcohol must be the solvent used to extract the herbal components. If you use glycerine, vinegar, only water (water used to dilute alcohol is fine), or any other menstruum (solvent) besides alcohol, your preparation is an extract rather than a tincture. Any type of liquor can be used, but many herbalists prefer a neutral spirit like vodka so the flavor of the herb can shine through.

Berries, leaves, roots, dried or fresh flowers, leaves, and other natural materials can be used to make them. Among them are dried mushrooms, vanilla beans, and stevia leaves.

## How Do You Use Tinctures

Tinctures are a type of dietary supplement that is liquid, concentrated, and shelf-stable. Similar to other herbal extracts, tinctures can be used to support a range of wellness objectives.

Since their effects will vary depending on the herb or herbs tinctured, the amount and frequency taken, and the individual ingesting them, it is advised that people seek the advice of a qualified medical professional for guidance on the most appropriate use for your specific needs.

In addition to being diluted in sparkling or black tea, tinctures can be consumed straight from the dropper. To give cocktail recipes flavor, some tinctures can be added.

Bowls made of ceramic and wood that contain dried herbs used to make tinctures are arranged on a table with light wood.

## Two Different Approaches to Herb Tincture.

**The Percolation Method**: Complicated But Simple.

If you enjoy hobbies that call for attention, accuracy, and specialized equipment (or if you require a finished tincture in a few days or less), the percolation method may be ideal for you.

Both methods can benefit from the general guidance on herb proportions and alcohol percentages provided in this post, but the percolation method requires a specific set of measurements and steps in order to be successful. Continue reading to get step-by-step instructions on how to make percolated herbal extracts from renowned herbalist Thomas Easley of the Eclectic School of Herbal Medicine.

## Though slow, the folk method is simple to use.

Unless you have some kind of convenient collapsible scale apparatus that fits in your processing kit, using the folk method is the best choice when making remedies in the forest, and it's great at home as well. This simple, practical, and efficient technique allows you to estimate your herb measurements without the need for any specialized tools.

You only need organic herbs, glass jars (either with a plastic lid or parchment paper/a sandwich bag to prevent the metal lid from corrosion), a knife or chopper, a metal funnel, cheesecloth, alcohol (sometimes referred to as a "menstruum" in tincture preparations), and amber glass dropper bottles.

The information in the following sections will also apply to the more expeditious percolation method of tincturing herbs, but it is written with the folk method in mind because it is more frequently used by home herbalists.

Let's get started with a few of the most important tincturing tips we've discovered over the years.

On a white background on a light wooden table, dried herbs and roots are displayed in mason jars.

13

Ratios of Fresh vs. Dried).

Start by putting the right amount of herbs in your tincturing container. Using insufficient amounts of the ingredients will lead to a weak tincture. Alcohol won't be able to extract all the medicinal plant compounds from your herbs if you use too much of it.

Different amounts of plant material and alcohol should be used, depending on what you are tincturing.

Below are a few guidelines for basic measurements.

**LEAVES and FRESH FLORALS.**

• Grind or finely chop a clean herb to release juice and reveal surface area.

• The herb should not fill the jar more than 2/3 of the way up.

• Pour as much alcohol as possible into the jar.

Plants should be completely enclosed!

• The herb should shake freely even though it appears to be in the jar in great abundance.


**FLOWERS and LEAVES that have been dried.**

• Use freshly chopped herbal material.

• Don't fill the jar with herb more than halfway or halfway.

• Pour booze into the entire jar.

• Completely enclose your plants!

## ALL FRESH ROOTS, BARKS, AND BERRIES.

• To release juice and reveal surface area, clean plants should be finely chopped or ground.

• Only use fresh roots, barks, or berries to fill the jar between 1/3 and 1/2 full

• To the brim with alcohol.

Completely encircle the plants!

• The herb should shake freely even though the jar appears to be full of it.


## DRIED ROOTS, BAKS, AND BERRIES.

• Make use of recently chopped herbal materials.

• Don't add dried berries, roots, or barks to the jar in amounts greater than 1/4 to 1/3.

• Pour enough alcohol to completely fill the jar.

• Enclose plants completely!

• Roots and berries will expand to twice their original size when reconstituted!

• Alcohol is being poured over herbs for tinctures in glass Mason jars on wooden tables against a white backdrop.


**Alcohol brand and strength.**
You must first fill your container with the proper quantity of plant material before adding a high-proof alcohol to make up the empty space. A high-quality, flavorless spirit like vodka or grain alcohol is preferred by many herbalists, though. Although most

spirits will function, they are not necessary. To achieve a lower alcohol content by volume, stronger alcohols can be diluted with distilled water.

The characteristics of the plant material being used will dictate the right alcohol strength for your tincture.

**Stronger isn't always better.**

As a general rule, you should match the alcohol strength of your tincture to the herb being used.

Between 40 and 50 percent of the alcohol by volume in 80 to 90 proof vodka.

• For tinctures, the "Standard" percentage range.

• Good for most dried herbs and fresh herbs that aren't overly juicy.

- Effective for removing water-soluble properties.

The alcohol by volume (ABV) ranges from 67.5% to 70% (made up of equal parts grain alcohol and vodka with proofs of 80 and 190).

- Removing the most flammable aromatic components.

- Beneficial for fresh herbs like lemon balm that have a high moisture content.

- Because of the higher alcohol content, more plant juices will be extracted.

190-proof grain alcohol has an alcohol content that ranges from 85% to 95% by volume.

• Beneficial for breaking down resins and gums but not necessary for the majority of plant material.

• Recuperates the aromatics and essential oils that are inextricably bound to the plant and difficult to evaporate.

• The use of botanicals other than gums and resins may result in a tincture that is difficult to take and will dehydrate the herbs if the alcohol content is this high.

## Where to Find Organic Grain Alcohol That Is Pure For Extracts.

When looking for high-quality alcohol to use with their herbal extracts, people frequently ask us for recommendations. If at all possible, we suggest visiting your local distillery (don't be afraid to ask for what you're looking for; they frequently will place special orders for you at no cost!). If shopping locally is not an option for you for this particular item, there are a number of online retailers who can help.

At-home apothecary concoctions, the following resources are suggested.

Distillers Fireside.

• The Organic Alcohol Co.

• A kitchen cleaner.

After being extracted, the tincture is being transferred to a new jar by being filtered through cheesecloth.

**Period of Tincture Extraction.**

Tinctures must have a lid on them while they are being extracted. Because some tinctures can actually melt plastic (especially those that contain aromatic herbs), we suggest using a standard metal canning jar lid with rim. If you plan to let your tincture macerate for at least six months, you might want to consider using parchment paper underneath the rim of the container before tightening it to prevent corrosion (a paper sandwich bag also works well). If you go this route, make sure there isn't any air between the liquid and the lid because too much air combined with the parchment can cause tinctures with insufficient alcohol content to rot.

Keep your tincture in a place that's dry, dark, and cool. Keep an eye on your alcohol intake and shake frequently. If any alcohol has evaporated and more alcohol needs to be added to the jar, make sure the herb is completely submerged. Herbs exposed to air may introduce mold and bacteria into your tincture. Give the mixture 6 to 8 weeks to extract.

• Placing Your Tinctures in Bottles.

• It's now time to squeeze!

A cobalt or amber glass bottle with a funnel should be covered with damp cheesecloth. Pour the tincture into the funnel, then watch it drip. then continue to twist and squeeze until you are unable to twist any longer.

Alternately, you could make a paste out of the herbs by pureeing them, and then strain the resulting liquid. If you keep the extracts in a dark, cool location, your tinctures might last for many years.

## Guidelines for Tincture Labeling.

Perhaps the most important step of all is the last one, labeling your creation.

Make sure to label each bottle completely after straining and bottling your tincture. You'll be thrilled to have this knowledge at your disposal the next time you tincture the same herb. Do not rely solely on your sense of taste or smell, regardless of how well-honed your organoleptic skills are.

Even the most seasoned herbalist may be misled by tinctures. You will undoubtedly end up with a dust-covered collection of useless mystery extracts if you skip this step.

What You Should Know and How to Use Herbal Tinctures.

Tinctures are concentrated herbal extracts created by soaking the bark, berries, leaves (fresh or dried), or roots of one or more plants in alcohol or vinegar.

The alcohol or vinegar draws out and concentrates the active elements of the plant parts into a liquid.

Tinctures, a common component of traditional herbal medicine for centuries, are heavily utilized.

Benefits of using a tincture.

Tinctures make it simple to consume the organic, health-improving chemicals found in some plants. Typically, they are easy and affordable to make at home.

It's estimated that 80% of people worldwide rely on herbal treatments like tinctures for at least some of their healthcare requirements, which is likely due in large part to how convenient they are to obtain.

Studies claim that the common tincture-making plants have health advantages.

Called chamomile, a flower.

Sources claim that chamomile is a plant that can be used to treat anxiety, mend wounds, and reduce inflammation.

Feverfew leaves. Historically, feverfew was used to lower fevers, but today it is mainly used to treat arthritis and ward off migraines. However, there are conflicting findings from studies on feverfew's ability to stop migraines. Some people insist it works, while others insist it doesn't. Recent research suggests that feverfew may be used to treat cancer, pain, and rosacea. Feverfew was tested in a mouse study as a possible treatment for anxiety and depression, and the results were promising.

(Root and cloves) garlic.

An analysis of a number of small and limited scientific studies suggested that garlic may be effective at lowering LDL (bad) and total cholesterol in small doses, but the findings were inconclusive.

Results of a subsequent analysis tended to be a little more conclusive.

They asserted that using garlic for more than two months reduced both total cholesterol and LDL cholesterol.

Currently, scientists are investigating garlic's potential as a cancer treatment.

Ginkgo leaf.

Ginkgo has been used for centuries to treat conditions ranging from asthma to tinnitus.

Recent scientific research has examined its potential to improve memory, prevent dementia, and improve brain function. Ginkgo contains chemicals that enhance the way brain cells function, claim studiesTrusted Source. The impact on how a person's brain functions in daily life is not, however, explained.

the ginseng plant's root. According to studies, ginseng may benefit the brain and immune system. It also suggests ginseng might be advantageous for people with diabetes.

Saw palmetto fruit is a fruit.

Saw palmetto has been used for many years to treat benign prostatic hypertrophy, but recent studies suggest that its effectiveness may not be as high as once believed.

Valerian, the root.

A small, constrained review of studies found that valerian root may improve the quality of your sleep.

There could be negative effects from tincture use.

Utilizing tinctures and other herbal remedies entails some risk. Even with plants whose health benefits have been scientifically proven, there is a chance of side effects, some of which are severe.

Consequences of taking medicine.

In some patients, herbal remedies and pharmaceuticals may interact.

As a consequence, this might lead to:.


• based on the medication.

• a problem with blood clotting.


• harm to the liver.

• the drug's increased effects.

• signs of an allergy.

It's possible to develop an allergy to some plants. A variety of responses are possible.

• fever.

• Itchiness.

• hives.

• redness.

• enlargement.

• an allergic reaction.

• a drop in blood sugar levels.

Diabetics should use caution when tinctures and other herbal remedies are used. Consuming certain plants, such as milk thistle, can result in dangerously low blood pressure.

Death.

Some plants, or parts of plants, are extremely toxic and should be avoided.

For instance, gingko leaves are a common herbal remedy. However, toxic gingko seeds should be avoided. They may cause convulsions or even cause death. Goldenseal is toxic in high doses.


Estrogen's side effects.

The milk thistle is one plant that may have estrogenic qualities. The possessors shouldn't take it.

• ovarian, breast, or uterine cancer.


• Endometriosis.

• ovarian fibroids.

• By increasing the body's estrogen levels, it might exacerbate these issues.

Digestive issues.

Some plants used in herbal remedies may cause these digestive issues:.

• bloating.

• indigestion.

• Diarrhea.

• gas.

• bloating.

• sickness.

• vertigo, sensitivity to light, and headache.

specific plants, such as St. John's wort can make you more sensitive to light if you take it in large doses. Vertigo and headaches are symptoms that some plants, like valerian, can cause.

Sleeplessness.

There are some plants that have stimulant properties that can keep you up at night.

## Under the tongue, the mixture burns

Burns or irritation are frequent side effects of some plant tinctures, most frequently appearing under the tongue.

For instance, goldenseal is well known for irritating the mouth's interior and the rest of the digestive system.

## Making a tincture.

Plants that are safe to use can be used to make tinctures at home. Herbs should be soaked in alcohol in a glass jar for the quickest and easiest way to make a tincture. Here is how:

- Locate the plant(s) you want to use. Make sure to only take the plant's safe to use parts.
- Finely chopped fresh leaves should fill a glass jar two-thirds to three-fourths of the way. Add bark, berries, or dried leaves and roots to the halfway mark. And fill it up one-fourth of the way with berries, dried roots, or bark.

- To completely cover the herbs in your glass jar, add grain alcohol with a 40–70% alcohol content.
- After placing a metal lid on top of the jar, cover it with parchment paper.
- Give it 6 to 8 weeks to rest.
- You should let your tincture drip through a cheesecloth that has been placed over a funnel.
- Your tincture is the liquid that has been strained.
- If you bottle it and keep it somewhere cool and dark, you can keep it for years.
- tincture preparation without the use of alcohol.
- No worries if you don't drink. Replace the alcohol in your tincture with white or apple cider vinegar

•

## Where to purchase tinctures

You can buy tinctures in most health food stores if you don't want to make your own. Before including tinctures in your daily healthcare routine, consult a physician.

Additionally, tinctures can be bought online.

## How to apply a tincture

Many tinctures are designed to be ingested orally while applying a small amount of liquid to the tongue using a dropper.

When using a tincture, only take the recommended dosage, which varies depending on things like:

- the concentration of the tincture
- you as a gender

- age and size of the body

It's important to take the time to educate yourself on the labels of tinctures you buy or look up the dosages for various plants online. Only the skin should be used with certain tinctures.

## The uses of well-known tinctures
We've already talked about some of the most well-known plants used in herbal remedies, like tinctures.

Particularly, some of the most well-liked tinctures at the moment are:

## The arnica tincture
Inflammatory skin conditions like rosacea are frequently treated with arnica tinctures.

According to research, there is little effectiveness and a chance of serious side effects like an allergic reaction.

## Benzoin-based tincture

When the tincture is inhaled as steam, benzoin has traditionally been used to treat mouth, throat, and other respiratory tract inflammation.

Studies, however, indicate a limited efficacy and the possibility of an allergic reaction.

## The iodine tincture

A reliable antiseptic is iodine tincture. It works well to stop infection on:

- cuts made externally
- burns
- scrapes

**Propolis tincture**

Propolis may have antibiotic, antifungal, and antiviral properties when applied topically, according to a review of the literature.

Some people assert that it can be used to strengthen the immune system, but science has not adequately supported those assertions.

**Elderberry tincture**

Anthocyanin, a potent antioxidant present in elderberries, is known to have anti-inflammatory properties. Elderberry tincture could possibly have an anti-inflammatory effect on the body.

## Turmeric tincture

The anti-inflammatory and antioxidant compoundcurcumin is found in turmeric.

It's possible that turmeric tinctures have a similar anti-inflammatory effect to curcumin, which appears to lessen knee pain in people with osteoarthritis.

## Tincture made from echinacea

The plant is effective at boosting the immune system, according to a review of the available research on echinacea.

Echinacea tincture is said to treat and prevent by those who practice herbal medicine when made from the leaves, stalk, and root.

- colds
- flus
- infections

Additionally, they assert that it can mend injuries.

## Cannabis tincture

Cannabidiol (CBD), a substance, is used to make cannabis tinctures.

## The advantages of mixing tinctures

It's simple, enjoyable, and frequently helpful to blend extracts. It might be easier to motivate yourself to take certain extracts if you combine them into a blend if you take them regularly together (for example, in the morning before work or at night before bed). Blends can also save a lot of room, which is particularly useful when you need plant support while traveling or on your morning commute. Blending can sometimes produce formulas that are more effective than the sum of their individual components because the dynamic qualities of the ingredients are emphasized by one another.

hand-dropping-amber-colored-liquid-tincture-into-vintage-green-glass-surrounded-by-sprigs-of-herbs-and-plants-and-glass-bottles-of-herbal-tincture-blends

## Safety Advice for Blending Herbs

Some herbs are only safe in very specific doses, carry the risk of herb-drug or herb-herb interactions, or may not be suitable for some populations (children, pregnant or nursing women, people with certain medical conditions, etc.). Only under the supervision of a qualified individual should these herbs be used medicinally. Other herbs, on the other hand, are well studied, widely beneficial, and well-tolerated, making them excellent choices for beginning blending projects.

The botanicals in our roster of single herb extracts have been chosen for their accessibility and safety. Although we don't think there are any unique safety precautions or contraindications that you might need to take into account when blending with our extract line, we do advise reading the Caution section on each extract's product page before adding it to your apothecary inventory

We focus on nervines, adaptogens, and digestives because their effects can frequently be felt shortly after consumption, making it simpler for a person to comprehend how they react to a new plant on a personal level—mentally, emotionally, physically, or spiritually. It might not be the right herb for you if an extract feels too potent or causes you any sort of discomfort. Nevertheless, some people experience an unpleasant strong reaction when taking an herb like valerian alone, but they enjoy it perfectly when combined in a formula. Prior to blending in bulk, we advise getting to know the specific formulas and individual herbs so that you can keep an eye out for any negative reactions and compare the effects of each against one another. alongside additional ingredients. If you're unsure, speak with a nearby herbalist for more advice

## Recipes for homemade herb tincture blends

We like to modify our favorite signature and traditional Chinese blends with one or two other herbs to highlight different aspects of the base formula and strengthen its effect. Our single herb extracts are amazing tools for easily adding flexibility to your home apothecary—which is why we use them so frequently ourselves. In order to create useful "secret menu" formulas that we don't currently pre-blend in our shop, we also combine individual extracts into straightforward blends.

Here are some of our favorite tweaks and mixtures that we've developed through home experiments, collaboration with friends, clients, and customers, and other sources. The ingredients for each modification are all available in our online shop, but please note that they are only intended for DIY projects. Close-up of blooming bright orange California poppy flowers growing outdoors. Feel free to modify, add to, and come up with fun new names whenever inspiration strikes.

## Five Flavor and Herb Formulas Have Had Modifications.

- Keep a positive attitude despite the hectic pre-holiday preparations with the "Positive Energy" mods
- Silk tree or passionflower extract is added to three parts of the Sustainable Energy formula
- During a stressful time, strengthen your physical and emotional resiliency with the "Vital Champion" mods.
- Ashwagandha or astragalus extract is added to the Mushroom Champion formula in 4:1

**Stay in School Mods:** Our adaptation of the TCM remedy "Jade Windscreen" for thwarting external health threats adds long-haul immune support to the acute action.

Add 2 tablespoons of Back to School formula and 1 tablespoon of reishi extract to cinnamon-ginger tea at the first sign of the sniffles for added support.

**"Moon Dance" Mod:** Use Chinese and Western herbs to treat the physical and psychological symptoms of PMS to make the start of your period a celebration rather than a trial.

1 part Elation formula plus 1 part Vitex extract (try our New Moon formula with vitex and blood-moving dong quai for extra cramp support if your PMS symptoms are more physical than emotional).

Resolve digestive upset caused by emotions like fear, worry, grief, or anger with the "Rectify Churn" mods.

## G in two parts

Add one part of the Holy Basil extract to the Feel Better or Rectify Qi formula.

Maintain your energy, concentration, and composure when working on projects that call for prolonged periods of focus and mental fortitude.

1 part of the Clarity formula plus 1 part of the Tian Wang Bu Xian Dan formula or Gui Pi Tang formula.

## Recipes for Single Herb Extract Blends

Take care of your mind and body's ability to remain calm with the "Stay Grounded" Blend, a mild nerve tonic.

1 part each of the extracts from California poppies, milky oats, and passionflower.

**"Sacred Balance" Blend:** With this complementary combination of adaptogenic, blood sugar-balancing, and spirit-calming botanicals, find a healthy middle ground on a number of levels.

- 2 parts Reishi extract plus 1 part Eleuthero extract from holy basil.

- With herbs that promote a sense of calm well-being and melodic elation, the "Bliss Balm" Blend makes it easier to experience joy.

- A cup of rosebud tea might benefit from the addition of 1 part of silk tree extract, 1 part of holy basil extract, and 1 part of lemon balm extract.

- Get relief from mild anxiety that occasionally manifests as jitters, agitation, irritability, or nervousness in crowds with the "Gimme Shelter" blend.

- Holy Basil extract is made up of two parts Holy Basil, one part Skullcap, and one part of a close-up of blossoming small purple Tulsi flowers and leaves growing outdoors

**Blending the herbs before tincturing**
There are times when we choose to combine herbs before extraction, producing a finished tincture that has the properties of several herbs right from the start. Making herbal

tinctures is outside the scope of this article, but we want readers to be aware that both approaches can be helpful for formulating, depending on the botanicals used and the desired result.

One benefit of creating pre-blended combination tinctures is that you can create a specific end formula all at once, as opposed to having to produce numerous single plant extracts and then blend them to create a finished product, when you have a specific formula in mind. This approach can be effective in terms of ingredient conservation as it reduces the possibility of having extra amounts of single plant extracts that may remain after blending and for which you may not have a clear use. Of course, blending your herbs before extraction makes it impossible to separate the components of the final formulation, which reduces your versatility.

We enjoy combining plants from our farm, Sunset Ranch, and those we've collected on foraging trips to make tinctures. We frequently combine some of our favorite fresh herbs into dependable combinations after bringing in a crop for use in Five Flavors Herbs products for our own use in our homes or clinics. For instance, the ingredients in our patented Skull Soother formula (skullcap, vervain, and feverfew) have a profound calming, relaxing, and soothing effect on headache discomfort. In the clinic, we frequently combine this collection of herbs with Bupleurum (chai hu) formulas to help activate and augment their effects for patients dealing with agitation associated with substance use or medication withdrawal, PMS, and a variety of psycho emotional and neurologic conditions.

## A guide to creating an herbal tincture.

To relieve your symptoms and treat any illnesses you may have, many herbs can be harvested and turned into "tinctures.". Making tinctures is surprisingly easy. How to make herbal tinctures from plants in your garden is provided here.

### What is an herbal tincture?

The most potent tinctures can be made from fresh herbs, and the process is very straightforward.

To extract and concentrate the medicinal constituents of herbs, which are molecules that plants produced for defense and that humans appropriated for our own medicinal use, herbs are steeped in high-proof ethyl alcohol (and occasionally vinegar).

Witch hazel is a plant used for natural first aid.

## How to Make Flavored Vinegars.
You can create a straightforward herbal salve for healing.

Most tinctures made from ethanol are intended to be taken internally. Liniments are only intended for external use and are made from tinctured herbal preparations. You can make them with oil, witch hazel, or rubbing alcohol (isopropyl).

Although you can tincture leaves or needles, flowers, roots, and barks—fresh or dried—I make mine primarily from fresh leaves that I gather from my gardens, lawns, and nearby wild places. As well as plantains that are overrunning the lawn and lemon balm that is beckoning to me from the herb garden, I'm gathering burdock flowers and leaves today.

**Positive qualities of tinctures.**
Medicinal plants can be smoked (so their medicinal components enter the body through the lungs) or brewed into teas or simmered into decoctions, mashed into poultices and salves, or extracted into tinctures depending on the illness being treated (or avoided). Tinctures are typically consumed internally, several times per day, a few drops at a time, frequently in tea or

juice. Some tinctures can be applied directly to wounds or skin infections.

**The benefits of tinctures over other herbal preparations are numerous.**

When compared to water extracts e.g Water extracts typically concentrate and extract more valuable medicinal compounds (e.g.,, ethanol). g. tisanes, teas, and infusions).

Because tinctures are so concentrated, they take effect quickly.

Alcohol tinctures created with ethanol that is at least 80 proof don't go bad and, when stored properly, keep their potency for a very long time. (While they can be used to flavor marinades and salad dressings, tinctures made with wine or vinegar won't be as effective at extracting active phytocompounds and won't last as long.

Tinctures are small and convenient for packing in a purse or travel bag.

## To start with

You'll need to learn something, preferably a lot, about the how, why, when, and dosage to use a particular plant tincture. Participate in workshops, read books and articles, and have conversations with regional herbalists.

You must be absolutely certain that the plant you intend to use has been correctly identified. Do invest in some field guides for wild plants or register for a workshop in your area to learn how to recognize them.

Only tincture plants that you are certain have not been treated with pesticides.

Plants gathered along highways or along the edges of fields used for industrial farming should not be used.


The necessary thing.

The plant parts you want to tincture. To stop the alcohol from being diluted by water, don't wash them. (Roots are an exception; you may wish to rinse or even lightly scrub them prior to chopping. If the plant parts are already wet, spread them out and gently blot them with a clean towel to dry them. Throw away any damaged or contaminated materials.

A bottle of 80 proof or higher ethyl alcohol. Many herbalists favor vodka because it is largely flavor, color, and odor neutral.

A glass container with an airtight lid.

Because alcohol tinctures are strong plant medicines that are only occasionally used, there is no need to make them in large bottles. Start out with small containers, such as emptied jam jars or pint canning jars.

A couple of tiny, dark bottles for the decanted tincture(s). Keep them in the dark to preserve their potency.

## Techniques for Making an Herbal Tincture.

• Leave delicate flowers and leaves whole; chop larger flowers, leaves, or roots. The plant material should be placed into the glass jar loosely, and then alcohol should be placed on top of it.

Cap the jar securely.

• A date should be written on the container.

• Indicate the specific plant parts that were tinctured as well as the type of alcohol used. For a month or more, place the jar in a cool, dark place. When necessary, add more alcohol to keep the plant materials submerged by shaking or stirring the mixture from time to time.

Use a clean piece of cheesecloth to strain the tincture into a glass or ceramic container, twisting the cloth to extract as much tincture as you can. Fill bottles made of dark glass with the tincture, and then tightly cap (or cork) each one. Each tincture needs to be identified, given a date, and kept in a cool, dark location.

• A tincture's concentration can be raised by removing the original plant matter and replacing it with fresh substance.

**Caveats.**

Like any other form of treatment, herbal remedies can have undesirable side effects. Learn all you can about an herb before attempting to use it. Your homemade tinctures don't offer a consistent "dose. Try a few drops of a new tincture in some warm water or tea as a starting point, and then gradually increase the dosage until the desired effects are experienced.

If you are pregnant, nursing, taking prescription medication, or you have a chronic illness, wait before starting an herbal remedy. Whenever you provide a doctor or dentist with information about you, mention whether you use herbs.

## What exactly is a tincture?

A tincture is a concentrated herbal extract dissolved in ethanol or vinegar.

These remedies have traditionally been used in Traditional Herbal Medicine to heal or prevent illness.

They are regarded as being incredibly efficient and easy to both make and use.

Selective components of one or more plants are prepared by soaking them in the liquid (typically alcohol), which is then removed after some time. The liquid that remains after the plant(s) used have released their properties is referred to as a tincture.

Tinctures are an essential component of many healing techniques used in traditional medicine all over the world because they are a remarkably simple way to administer herbal remedies.

# What are the benefits of tinctures

Applying tinctures is easy.

They are not difficult to swallow, unlike a capsule, and do not require multiple daily preparations like a tea.

Because many herbs don't make particularly good tea, people are more likely to choose tinctures when selecting an herbal remedy.

Tinctures typically come in tiny dropper bottles, making them portable for dosing throughout the day.

A few drops in a cup of tea or water are all that is needed.

Depending on the needs, this might take place just once or several times throughout the day.

Bottle with a dropper for the tincture.

Taking propolis, ginseng, or echinacea tinctures can boost the immune system.

They should be taken once daily for two to three weeks if our only goal is to get ready for the coming winter. On the other hand, if we experience symptoms and want to speed up our body's recovery, we take them several times per day for two to three days.

**Important details:**

Generally speaking, it is not advisable to use herbal tinctures continuously all year long.

Unless otherwise specified, there must be a break after a period of 4-6 weeks of consistent use.

# How to Quickly and Simply Make a Homemade Herbal Tincture.

How does it operate?

Homemade herbal tinctures are typically made by soaking the selected herb(s) in alcohol at a ratio ranging from 1:1 (herb to alcohol) to 1:10, depending on the desired potency and the recommended dosage of those particular herbs.

When using dried herbs, the typical ratio is 1:4 (one part dried herb to four parts alcohol), while the typical ratio when using fresh herbs is 1:1.

After 4 to 8 weeks, the medicinal properties of the herbs have dissolved into the liquid.

After the plant material has been strained and removed, the liquid is usually poured into tiny, labeled, dark glass bottles with dropper tops.

We concentrate on nervines, adaptogens, and digestives because they frequently have effects that are noticeable soon after consumption, making it easier for a person to understand how they respond to a new plant on a personal level—mentally, emotionally, physically, or spiritually. If an extract feels too potent or causes you any kind of discomfort, it might not be the herb for you. However, some people react strongly and unfavorably to an herb like valerian when taken alone, but they love it when it's combined with other ingredients in a formula. We suggest familiarizing yourself with the specific blends and individual herbs before blending large quantities so that you can watch out for any adverse reactions and contrast the effects of each herb with one another. with additional ingredients. Consult a local herbalist for more information if you're unsure.

## Herbal tincture blends made at home with recipes.

With the addition of one or two other herbs, we like to alter our favorite signature and traditional Chinese blends in order to emphasize particular qualities of the base mixture and enhance its impact. The reason we use them so frequently ourselves is because our single herb extracts are incredible tools for quickly adding flexibility to your home apothecary. Additionally, we blend separate extracts into simple blends to produce useful "secret menu" formulas that are not currently pre-blend in our shop.

**There Have Been Modifications To Five Flavor And Herb Formulas.**

With the "Positive Energy" mods, you can remain upbeat despite the hectic pre-holiday preparations.

The Sustainable Energy formula calls for the addition of three parts of silk tree or passionflower extract.

With the "Vital Champion" mods, you can increase your physical and psychological resilience during a difficult time.

The Mushroom Champion formula includes a 4:1 addition of ashwagandha or astragalus extract.

Stay in School Mods: We have added long-term immune support to the acute action of the TCM remedy "Jade Windscreen" for fending off external health threats.

When the sniffles start, make a cup of cinnamon-ginger tea with 2 tablespoons of Back to School formula and 1 tablespoon of reishi extract.

Use Chinese and Western herbs to treat PMS's physical and psychological symptoms to make the beginning of your period a celebration rather than a hardship.

For additional cramp support, try our New Moon formula with vitex and blood-moving dong quai if your PMS symptoms are more physically than emotionally based.

Using the "Rectify Churn" mods, you can soothe digestive distress brought on by feelings of fear, worry, grief, or anger.

**Two parts of G.**

To the Feel Better or Rectify Qi formula, add one part of the Holy Basil extract.

When working on tasks that demand sustained periods of focus and mental fortitude, keep your energy, concentration, and composure.

1 part of the Gui Pi Tang formula and 1 part of either the Tian Wang Bu Xian Dan formula or the Clarity formula.

**Recipes for Single-Herb Extract Blends.**
• Use the mild nerve tonic "Stay Grounded" Blend to take care of your mind and body's capacity for composure.

• 1 part each of the extracts from passionflower, milky oats, and California poppies.

• "Sacred Balance" Blend: Reach a balanced middle ground on a number of levels with this complementary mixture of adaptogenic, blood sugar-balancing, and spirit-calming botanicals.

• 2 parts of reishi extract and 1 part of eleuthero from holy basil.

• The "Bliss Balm" Blend facilitates joy by containing herbs that foster feelings of calm well-being and melodic elation.

• A cup of rosebud tea might benefit from the addition of one part each of the extracts from the silk tree, the holy basil plant, and the lemon balm plant.

• Use the "Gimme Shelter" blend to get relief from mild anxiety that occasionally shows up as jitters, agitation, irritability, or nervousness in crowds.

• A close-up of blossoming small purple Tulsi flowers and leaves growing outdoors is used to make the holy basil extract, which is composed of two parts holy basil, one part skullcap, and one part.

Prior to tincturing, the herbs are blended.

In some cases, we decide to combine the herbs before extracting them, resulting in a finished tincture that has the properties of several herbs right away. Although making herbal tinctures is beyond the scope of this article, we want readers to be aware that both methods can be useful for formulating, depending on the botanicals used and the desired outcome.

When you have a specific end formula in mind, one advantage of producing pre-blended combination tinctures is that you can create it all at once as opposed to having to produce numerous single plant extracts and then blend them to create a finished product. As it lessens the possibility of having extra amounts of individual plant extracts that may remain after blending and for which you may not have a clear use, this strategy can be effective in terms of ingredient conservation. Of course, blending your herbs before extraction makes it impossible to separate the ingredients of the final formulation, which limits your adaptability.

To help you manage your symptoms and recover from any illnesses you may have, many herbs can be harvested and turned into "tinctures.". Making tinctures is surprisingly easy. Here's how to make herbal tinctures from plants in your garden.

## SINGLE HERB EXTRACT BLEND RECIPES

Use the mild nerve tonic "Stay Grounded" Blend to take care of your mind and body's capacity for composure.

Milky oats, passionflower, and California poppy extracts, each in one part.

Find a healthy middle ground on various levels with the help of the adaptogenic, blood sugar-balancing, and spirit-calming botanicals that make up the "Sacred Balance" Blend.

1 part Eleuthero extract from holy basil and 2 parts Reishi extract.

The "Bliss Balm" Blend makes it simpler to feel joy because it contains herbs that foster feelings of calm well-being and melodic elation.

One part each of the extracts from the silk tree, holy basil, and lemon balm may be added to a cup of rosebud tea for added flavor.

The "Gimme Shelter" blend will help you cope with mild anxiety that occasionally appears as jitters, agitation, irritability, or nervousness in crowds.

A close-up of blossoming tiny purple Tulsi flowers and leaves growing outdoors makes up one part of the Holy Basil extract, which is composed of two parts Holy Basil, one part Skullcap, and one part.

prior to tincturing, the herbs are blended.

There are times when we decide to combine herbs before extraction, creating a finished tincture that has the properties of several herbs right from the start. Although making herbal tinctures is beyond the scope of this article, we want readers to be aware that both methods can be useful for formulating, depending on the botanicals used and the desired outcome.

When you have a specific end formula in mind, one advantage of producing pre-blended combination tinctures is that you can create it all at once as opposed to having to produce numerous single plant extracts and then blend them to create a finished product. This strategy can help preserve ingredients because it lessens the possibility of having extra amounts of single plant extracts that might remain after blending and for which you might not have a clear use. It goes without saying that blending your herbs before extraction makes it impossible to separate the ingredients of the finished product, which limits your versatility.

We enjoy combining plants from our farm, Sunset Ranch, and those we've collected on foraging trips to make tinctures. After harvesting a crop to use in Five Flavors Herbs products for our own use in our homes or clinics, we frequently combine some of our favorite fresh herbs into dependable combinations. For instance, the ingredients in our patented Skull Soother formula (skullcap, vervain, and feverfew) have a significant calming, relaxing, and soothing effect on headache discomfort. For patients dealing with agitation brought on by substance use or medication withdrawal, PMS, and a variety of psycho emotional and neurologic conditions, we frequently combine this collection of herbs with Bupleurum (chai hu) formulas in the clinic to help activate and augment their effects.

## A guide to creating an herbal tincture

To relieve your symptoms and treat any illnesses you may have, many herbs can be harvested and made into "tinctures.". Tinctures are surprisingly simple to make. Here's how to use plants from your garden to make herbal tinctures.

## This is what an herbal tincture is

Fresh herbs make the most potent tinctures, and making them is incredibly simple.

To extract and concentrate the medicinal components of herbs, which are molecules that plants produced for defense and that humans appropriated for our own medicinal use, the herbs are steeped in high-proof ethyl alcohol (and occasionally vinegar).

## Witch hazel, a plant used for first aid and natural remedies

**Flavored Vinegars:** How to Make Them.

A Simple Herbal Salve for Healing can be made.

Ether tinctures are typically intended for internal consumption. Liniments are herbal preparations that have been tinctured and are only meant to be applied externally. They can be produced using oil, witch hazel, or rubbing alcohol (isopropyl).

Although you can tincture leaves or needles, flowers, roots, and barks—fresh or dried—I make mine primarily from fresh leaves that I gather from my gardens, lawns, and nearby wild places.

## Tinctures' positive attributes

Depending on the illness being treated (or avoided), medicinal plants can be brewed into teas or simmered into decoctions, mashed into poultices and salves, smoked (so their medicinal components enter the body through the lungs), or extracted into tinctures. Tinctures are typically taken internally, a few drops at a time, several times per day, frequently in tea or juice. To treat wounds or skin infections, some tinctures can be applied directly.

Over other herbal formulations, tinctures have a number of advantages.

Comparatively to water extracts (e.g. ethanol), water extracts typically extract and concentrate more valuable medicinal compounds. g. infusions, tisanes, and teas).

Tinctures are effective quickly because they are so concentrated.

Alcohol tinctures made with ethanol that is at least 80 proof do not go bad and, when stored properly, retain their potency for a very long time. (While they can be enjoyed in marinades and salad dressings, tinctures made with wine or vinegar won't extract as many active phytocompounds and won't last as long.

Tinctures are compact and simple to tuck into a purse or travel bag.

Before you begin.

You'll need to learn something, preferably a lot, about the how, why, when, and dosage to use a specific plant tincture. Attend workshops, read books and articles, and speak with local herbalists.

You must be absolutely certain that the plant you intend to use has been accurately identified. Do purchase some field guides for wild plants or sign up for one of the available workshops in your area to learn how to identify them.

Only tincture plants that you are certain have not received pesticide treatment.

Use should not be made of plants gathered near roadside or at the edges of fields used for commercial farming.

**What is required**

Parts of the plant that you intend to tincture. Don't wash them to prevent water from diluting the alcohol. (Roots are an exception; you might want to rinse or even lightly scrub them before chopping. If the plant parts are already wet, spread them out and gently blot them with a clean towel to dry them off. Discard any contaminated or broken materials.

a bottle of ethyl alcohol with an 80 proof or higher. Due to its largely neutral flavor, color, and odor, vodka is preferred by many herbalists.

a container made of glass with a secure lid. Making an alcohol tincture doesn't require using big bottles because it is only used sparingly—a tincture is a potent plant medicine. Start with small containers like empty jam or pint canning jars or pint canning jars.

For storing the decanted tincture(s),a few tiny, dark bottles. They retain more potency when kept in the dark.

## Traditional herbal remedies for healing

An old form of medicine that is still used today is Traditional Chinese Medicine (TCM). Shennong Ben Cao Jing, one of

TCM's most revered lists of healing plants, is one of the oldest herbal texts. The content of the text is attributed to ShenNong, a legendary healer who is believed to have lived around 2500 BCE, even though the written version of the text was recorded around 250 CE (Common Era, formerly AD). Whether ShenNong existed or not has been questioned, but the herbal remedies and uses for which ShenNong is credited have been passed down through centuries of oral tradition until the Chinese classic was compiled and recorded. The Shennong Ben Cao Jing includes minerals, herbs, woods, animals, fruits, and vegetables in its list of healing substances. Among the herbs mentioned are Mung Beans, Ginseng, Ling ZhiReishi, Ginger, and other contemporary herbal heroes.

Ayurveda was developing as a medical system in India at the same time.

In Sanskrit, the word "Ayurveda" means "Science of Life".

Yoga, meditation, astrology, and herbalism are all incorporated into the ancient medical system known as Ayurveda, which dates back to 3300 BCE. The Yajur Veda, Rig Veda, Sam Veda, and Atharva Veda are four knowledge collections that form the foundation of ayurvedic therapeutic systems. The Ayurvedic practice of using plants and botanicals is described in each of the Vedas. In order to achieve balance, ayurveda links plants to elements and the elements to bodily doshas. The primary Ayurvedic herbs turmeric and holy basil have long served as an inspiration for New Chapter formulations.

# The 18th century saw the use of herbs

According to legend, the 15th to the 17th centuries marked the height of herbalism. Having been translated from Latin and Greek, herbal books were now being made available in English. Grete Herball, which appeared in 1526, was one of the first herbal books to be translated into English. The first English book on herbalism, Banckes' Herbal, which was published in 1525, came before this. It is significant to note that Richard Banckes published Banckes' Herbal; the author is unknown. (There is some debate as to which book was published first; each has been cited as having been published in either 1525 or 1526, depending on the source. (A digital version of Banckes' Herbal can be found online at the U. S. It mentions Rosemary, Lavender, Mint, and Chamomile, which are still used by New Chapter today as therapeutic herbal ingredients, so it's worth a look.

**Elderberry products by New Chapter**
This introduces Nicolas Culpeper, who was alive from 1616 to 1654. Culpeper, an English herbalist, botanist, and doctor, wrote The Complete Herbal, a comprehensive tome on herbal and pharmacological knowledge. Culpeper had a reputation for being a rebel, much like Hippocrates. During a time when medicine was primarily used by the aristocracy, he worked as a herbalist for the general public. This indicated that he was despised by the medical profession at the time. More ancient practices like

bloodletting were frowned upon by Culpeper.

The fact that women were frequently tasked with gathering roots and taking care of their families contributed significantly to herbalism's rise to popularity in the American colonies. Native Americans' use of plant-based medicine was essential in assisting the Europeans in making the transition to the American landscape.

When discussing the continued practice of herbalism in the United States, it is important to acknowledge the role of Black, Indigenous, and people of color in the country. The ability to use plants to support healing was a tradition passed down among oppressed people in order to have access to medicine. Some states outlawed the teaching or study of herbal medicine by slaves in the middle of the 18th century.

Harriet Tubman, a well-known Black herbalist, is credited with using her knowledge of plants to help passengers on the Underground Railroad. George Washington Carver (1864–1943), an agricultural scientist and prolific inventor, is another significant figure in the history of herbs. Carver was a pioneer in promoting future herbalism and soil health through his work on nitrogen-rich plants like soybeans and peanuts, soil restoration, crop rotation, yield enhancement, and the development of natural pesticides.

# Herbalism of Today and Tomorrow

From the Salem Witch Trials' botanical associations with witchcraft to the way medical students are taught about herbalism, the idea that herbalism is a taboo subject has appeared numerous times throughout history. The American Medical Association (AMA) established the Council on Medical Education in 1904, which had a significant impact on the development of herbalism in North America. The American Medical Association (AMA) sought to impose strict requirements on medical schools in regards to medical education. They closed down schools that couldn't live up to their standards. More than half of American medical schools closed or merged with major universities between 1910 and 1935. Because doing so would result in their losing their accreditation—which was essential for their survival—these schools were not permitted to provide instruction in homeopathy, naturopathy, chiropractic, or osteopathic practice. It was clear that teaching about the therapeutic use of herbs was not a priority in medical curricula.

## Emergency Medicine

An emergency situation with regard to medicine is anaphylaxis.

After taking a tincture, if you or anyone else experiences difficulty breathing or swallowing, dial 911 and head to the closest emergency room.

## A reduction in blood sugar

The use of tinctures and other herbal remedies should be done with caution by people with diabetes.

Some plants, such as milk thistle, can cause dangerously low blood pressure.

## Death

- Avoid using certain plants or plant parts because they can be extremely toxic
- Gingko leaves are one popular herbal treatment, as an illustration
- Gingko seeds are poisonous, so it's crucial to stay away from them
- They may result in seizures and even death
- High doses of goldenseal are also toxic

## Effects of esters

Some plants, including milk thistle, may have estrogenic properties.

- Anyone who has: shouldn't take it.
- ovarian, breast, or uterine cancer.
- endometriosis.
- The uterine fibroids.
- These problems could get worse because it could raise the body's estrogen levels.
- digestive disorders

The following gastrointestinal problems could be brought on by certain plants used in herbal remedies:

- Bloating
- constipation.
- diarrhea.
- gas.

- heartburn.
- nausea.

**Nausea, light sensitivity, and headache.**

Some plants, like the St. Taking large doses of John's wort can make you more sensitive to light. Dizziness and headaches can be brought on by other plants, like valerian.

**Sleeplessness**

Certain plants that are stimulating can keep you up at night.

Tincture causes tongue burn.

Burns or irritation are frequent side effects of some plant tinctures, most frequently appearing under the tongue.

For instance, goldenseal has a reputation for irritating the mouth's interior and the rest of the digestive system.

## The best way to make tinctures without alcohol

No problem if you're not a drinker. Replace the alcohol in your tincture with white or apple cider vinegar.

You can buy tinctures in the majority of health food stores if you don't want to make your own. Before including tinctures in your medical regimen, consult a doctor.

Online shopping is another option for tinctures.

**A tincture's recommended use**
Many tinctures can be ingested orally by drizzling a small amount of liquid onto the tongue with a dropper.

When using a tincture, only take the recommended dosage, which varies depending on things like:

**The potency of the tincture**

- your sex.
- Age and physical size.

It's crucial to take the time to educate yourself about the recommended tincture dosages for various plants online or on the label of the tinctures you buy. Some tinctures can only be applied topically.

## The uses of well-known tinctures

We've already talked about some of the most well-known plants used in herbal remedies, including tinctures.

Particularly, the following tinctures are some of the most well-liked ones right now:.

## Arnica tincture

Rosacea and other inflammatory skin conditions are frequently treated with arnica tinctures. Limited efficacy and the possibility of serious side effects, such as an allergic reaction, are shown by research.

## The benzoin tincture

When inhaled as steam, benzoin tincture has traditionally been used to treat inflammation of the mouth, throat, and other respiratory passages.

## The iodine tincture

An effective antiseptic is iodine tincture. It can be utilized to stop infection on:

- cuts on the outside.
- burns.
- scrapes.

## Propolis tincture

Propolis may have antibiotic, antifungal, and antiviral properties when applied topically, according to a review of the literature.

Some people assert that it can be used to strengthen the immune system, but science has not adequately supported those assertions.

## Elderberry Tincture

Anthocyanin, a potent antioxidant found in elderberries, is known to have anti-inflammatory properties. Elderberry tincture might have an anti-inflammatory effect on the body.

## Turmeric tincture

The anti-inflammatory and antioxidant compound curcumin is found in turmeric.

It's possible that turmeric tinctures have a similar anti-inflammatory effect to how curcumin appears to lessen knee pain in people with osteoarthritis.

## Echinacea tincture

Echinacea is effective at boosting the immune system, according to a review of the research.

People who use herbal medicine assert that echinacea tincture made from the leaves, stalk, and root can treat and prevent:

- colds.
- flus.
- infections.
- They also assert that it can mend injuries

## Cannabis oil for tincture

A substance called cannabidiol (CBD) is used to make cannabis tinctures.

# How to Select High Quality Herbs and Herbal Treatments

On the market, not all herbal treatments work equally well. Use these indicators to confirm that the herbs and herbal medicine preparations you are purchasing are of the highest caliber.

The effectiveness of herbal medicines is influenced by a variety of elements, including growing conditions, the right time to harvest, the plant parts used, storage, contamination, and freshness.

This article will help you choose high-quality herbal medicines by examining all factors, from the growth of the plant to its preparation in medicine, whether you are purchasing dried herbs in bulk, small-batch preparations, or manufactured herbal products. The best source for learning about the quality of herbal preparations is speaking with your local herbalist or medicine maker. Some of these criteria may be listed on a label, while others will be more challenging to find.

## 1. Opt for the appropriate herb

Do your research or speak with a herbalist first. Herbs don't all have the same effects on people, and some can be dangerous for people with certain conditions or while taking medications. Prior to purchasing herbal remedies, it's critical to select the right herb, understand which plant parts contain the desired medicine, and determine the best preparation method for your requirements.

Various therapeutic uses can be made of the plant's various parts. You would need to choose the right plant and the right plant part to get the right medicine, for instance, stinging nettle roots and leaves both contain an anti-inflammatory compound, but only the roots contain the steroid-like compounds.

## 2. Contaminants don't affect plants

Herbs used for medicinal purposes should be sustainably wildcrafted or grown organically in a clean environment. Herbs that have been wildcrafted ought to be harvested in a tidy area away from pollution-causing sources like traffic. Has the area been sprayed with herbicides like glyphosate?

Look for USDA certification, wildcrafted products, or other statements of commitment to chemical-free agriculture when purchasing plants from North

America. The phrase "Grown and cultivated without chemicals" may appear on the label, indicating that the product was grown and cultivated without the use of pesticides, chemical fertilizers, herbicides, genetically modified organisms (GMOs), synthetic chemicals, irradiation, or chemical sterilization.

## 3. At their prime, plants are harvested

To obtain the most effective medicine, specific plant parts should be harvested at specific growth stages.

Pre-flowering in the spring is the typical time to gather leaves. The entire plant is harvested while it is in flower if all aerial parts are used.

Flowers are picked as soon as they open, before the wind or other pollinators remove the pollen.

With a few exceptions, such as milky oat seeds, which are harvested when the seed is still green and not fully ripe, most seeds are harvested when they are ripe.

Following the fall aerial part's demise, roots are typically harvested.

To get the most therapeutic benefit from high-quality herbs, they are harvested at their prime.

## 4. The medicine contains only the plant parts that are the strongest

The mere fact that a plant is regarded as medicinal does not imply that the entire plant is therapeutically useful. For instance, the flower head and a few of the leaves that encircle the flower are the only aerial parts of red clover that are medicinal. The medicine will be less effective if the product label reads "cut and sifted," which means the entire plant was used. Search for items with the word "blossom" on them.

## Preparation

It's a Reputable Company That Provides the Herbs.

When buying herbs, look for reputable, long-running businesses that understand their niche and have a solid track record. The saying "you get what you pay for" is frequently accurate. By substituting or including less expensive herbs in a preparation, adulterated herbal products can reduce their effectiveness.

Companies that process bulk dried herbs imported from abroad may use herbs that were exposed to radiation or fumigation during transport.

If the herbs are wild-crafted, the business must also state that it adheres to a sustainable harvesting policy.

## The Dose and Preparation are Correct for the Herb

Products made from prepared herbs are not all created equal, even with the best ingredients. The following are some things to watch out for in various preparations.

- Herbs that have been dried.

- Use your senses to help you select dried herbs

Herbs that are high quality should closely resemble the fresh plant in terms of color, texture, fragrance, and flavor. Longer-lasting freshness is correlated with larger pieces.

In order to extract the desired medicinal components for tinctures, the alcohol strength must be high enough, and the proportion of plant to alcohol must be suitable for the dose.

Herbs are steeped in a solution of alcohol and water known as the menstruum to create tinctures. The majority of herbal tinctures can be made with alcohol strengths between 25 and 40 percent, but some constituents, particularly resins, need a higher alcohol concentration to be extracted.

For instance, at least 70% of usnea must be consumed to reap the benefits of its antibacterial properties. Calendula can be extracted at lower percentages for some medicinal purposes, but it needs to be extracted at 90% to release the anti-fungal components from the resins.

The marc is the botanical component of a tincture. A skilled herbalist will be able to determine whether a plant should be dried or used fresh for tinctures.

The ratio of plant to liquid (marc to menstruum) indicates the tincture's potency on the bottle.

A ratio of 1:1 denotes an equal mix of plant and liquid.

A 1:5 tincture has 1 part plant matter and 5 parts liquid by weight, where the first

number represents the plant material and the second number represents the liquid. So, for instance, a 1:2 tincture is significantly stronger than a 1:5, etc. As a result, you would need to purchase less medication in order to receive the same dose. When comparing herbal tincture prices, it's important to keep in mind that the strength of the tincture should be reflected in the cost.

On the label of glycerites, which are water-glycerine preparations, there should also be a ratio that indicates the plant-to-glycerine ratio.

## Other Items

Here are some additional things to take into account when buying herbal products because herbal preparations can vary greatly.

## Are all active and inactive ingredients listed?

Some products may have a high proportion of safe ingredients or weaker herbs, so ask the seller if they include fillers.

When does it become invalid?

Is the scientific name of the plant and the plant part used on the label?

## The goods are brand-new

And last but not least, even the best herbs and herbal remedies don't last a lifetime. Due to the alcohol content, tinctures have a very long shelf life, but other preparations like glycerites, salves, and dried or powdered herbs have a shorter shelf life.

Dried herbs have a range of shelf lives. To avoid receiving dried herbs that have spent a long time on a shelf, buy from stores with a high turnover rate and place frequent orders. When compared to ground or powdered herbs, whole herbs last longer. In general, dried leaves and flowers last a year and dried roots, seeds, and barks up to two years.

The shelf life of herbal preparations is influenced by the longevity of the solvent used to extract the medication, i.e. the amount of glycerin, honey, vinegar, oil, and

other ingredients there is, as well as how easily bacteria will flourish in the dish. In contrast to honeys and vinegars, which go bad as a result of the growth of microbes, oil-based preparations are more likely to go bad due to rancidity, or oxidation. Product expiration dates should be checked. Glycerites can last up to three years in products without an expiration date, and syrups and vinegars can keep for about a year in the refrigerator.

In general, medicines will be most potent when they are derived from healthy plants that are harvested at the proper time of year and from the appropriate plant parts for the desired medicine.

You'll always get the best herbal medicine if you keep these factors in mind the next time you buy herbs. As you can see, it can be

tempting to purchase less expensive herbs or medications, but you might not get what you pay for if you do. Knowing local herbalists is the best way to purchase high-quality herbs and herbal remedies. Many herbalists produce their medicines in small batches, and they will be able to answer any questions you may have regarding the ingredients, process, and source. Even though buying locally is always preferable, they will know which brands to order from if they don't manufacture their own medications.

## Herbal remedies' toxicological risks

Patients with cancer, those suffering from chronic illnesses, and the general public, including children and teenagers, are using alternative medicines (AMs) more frequently. Through the Internet, the media,

publications, and friends, the general public is exposed to AMs. Well-known examples of AMs include herbal medicine, traditional Chinese medicine, homeopathy, naturopathic medicine, acupuncture, chiropractic, and Ayurvedic medicine. Some of the less well-known types include energy medicine, magnetic field therapy, aromatherapy, and oxygen therapy. Only a small amount of exposure to AMs occurs during medical school. The potential risks that AMs could present to their patients must be understood by doctors. The potential toxicity of herbal remedies is briefly discussed in the current committee note. It does not take into account their therapeutic effects, many of which have not been proven through randomized clinical trials.

## Why Is Quality Control Essential?

The active ingredient's concentration may differ depending on the plant part used (root, stem, leaf, or fruit). The concentration of the active ingredients may also be impacted by the harvesting season. Products harvested in the winter and summer, for instance, differ from one another. The use of potentially toxic plants in manufacturing has been reported to occur, and misidentification of plants has been reported.

A variety of herbal medicine formulations contain toxic plants.

Several plants have incorrect labels.

For instance, Periplocasepium was used in place of ginseng in a case where a baby was born with hirsutism after the mother consumed the product. Herbs have been

119

found to contain other contaminants like lead, arsenic, mercury, aflatoxin, mycobacterium, penicillium, coliforms, salmonella, candida, earthworms, and blister beetles.